The Art of
Reflexology

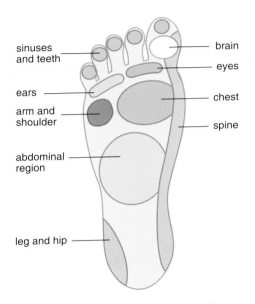

sinuses and teeth

brain

eyes

ears

chest

arm and shoulder

spine

abdominal region

leg and hip

The Art of Reflexology

Mapping the Sole

Nancy Arnott

Ariel Books

Andrews McMeel Publishing

Kansas City

www.andrewsmcmeel.com

Photographs on pp. 6, 8, 10, 23, 24, 29, 32, 35, 36, 40, 42, 48, 51, 56, 59, 62, 64-65, 71, 72, 74, 77, 79 © Carlton Books; pp.17, 26 courtesy International Institute of Reflexology, St. Petersburg, FL; artwork pp. 2,18, 46 by Mary Carnahan; p.66 © Koren Trygg.

ISBN: 0-8362-5223-3

Library of Congress Catalog Card Number: 97-74528

Contents

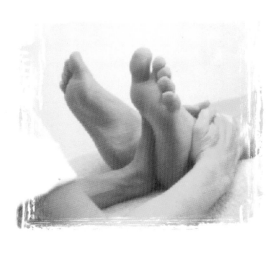

Introduction

Reflexology is the art of promoting overall well-being by manipulating the body's extremities—most commonly the feet, although some reflexologists also work with the hands and the ears. Like other forms of bodywork, such as massage and acupressure, reflexology is gaining popularity in the

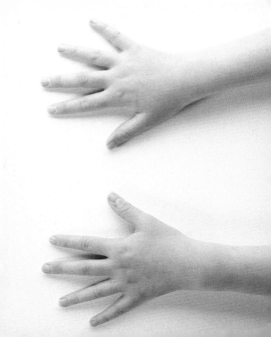

United States. It especially appeals to those interested in getting in touch with their bodies from head to toe, and enhancing their well-being at the same time.

This book is intended to satisfy the reader's curiosity about the practice of reflexology and its traditions, not to prescribe treatments for specific complaints. If you suffer from any medical problem, promptly consult your physician for advice.

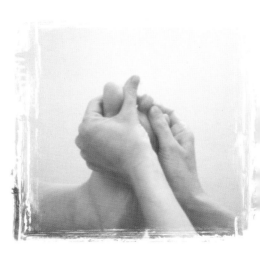

What Is Reflexology?

Reflexology is more than just a form of foot massage. It is a technique based on the theory that each part of the body is linked to a specific zone on the feet which, when manipulated by a reflexologist, stimulates a flow of vital energy to that corresponding body part. When you look at your own feet, you probably just see two bony appendages. But to a reflexologist's eyes, your feet display a complex map of all the organs and systems of your body. Using this map, the reflexologist can address discomfort or blocked energy in each body part by manipulating the appropriate points on the feet.

Historians haven't been able to establish exactly when and where reflexology got started, but they believe it originated in China around the same time as acupuncture. Both life-enhancing arts are believed to have their roots in a treatment system based on pressure points that was practiced in China and India possibly as long as five thousand years ago. Egyptians may also have

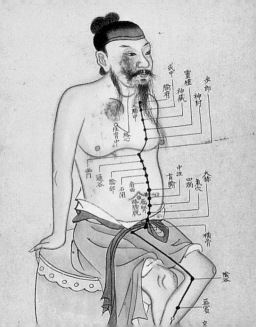

been among the earliest reflexologists: A painting from the year 2330 B.C. on the wall of the tomb of Ankhmahor in Saqqara, Egypt, depicts a physician administering what we would today call a reflexology treatment.

Reflexology was reborn in the West in the 1890s, when a German physician, Dr. Alfons Cornelius, developed the concept of applying massage techniques to specific "reflex zones" of the body to relieve pain. This notion was brought to the United States by Dr. William Fitzgerald, an American surgeon who found that he could perform minor surgical procedures less painfully if pressure was applied to specific reflex points on the patient's body, using elastic bands or small clamps. In 1917 Fitzgerald and a colleague, Dr. Edwin Bowers, published a

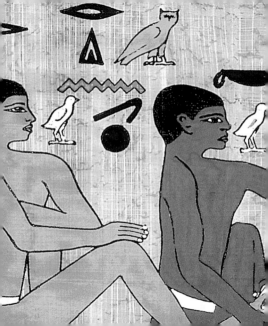

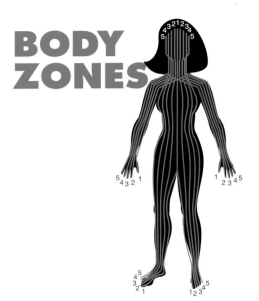

BODY
ZONES

book called *Zone Therapy*, which divided the body, including the feet, into ten zones and explained how treatment of one part of the body could affect other parts within that same zone.

Another American physician, Dr. Joseph Riley, was so impressed by Fitzgerald's ideas that he incorporated zone therapy into his practice. Eunice Ingham, a physiotherapist who worked with Riley, expanded on zone therapy's principles to develop the theories of modern reflexology in the 1930s. Over the next thirty years she refined its techniques and devised the detailed foot maps still used today. She also spread the word about this infant art by traveling across the United States, lecturing to health practitioners and laypeople alike, and writing the first books about reflexology.

Legitimate reflexologists do not promote themselves as medical practitioners or claim to be able to diagnose or cure illness. They do, however, believe that by encouraging relaxation and allowing vital energy to flow freely through the body, reflexology can enhance the body's own healing ability.

Potential benefits include:

- relieving everyday stress;
- improving circulation by keeping blood flowing freely to all parts of the body;
- facilitating the removal of toxins and waste products from the body;
- restoring balance, keeping all areas of the body working together;

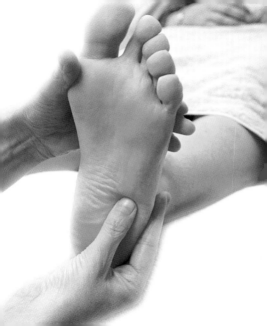

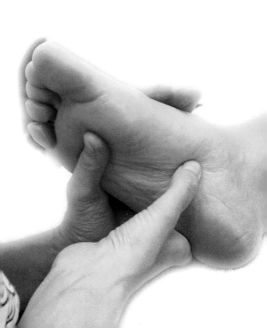

•increasing energy by relaxing the body and opening up its energy pathways;

•strengthening the immune system.

Treating the body as an integrated organism and bringing it into perfect balance is the reflexologist's goal. For this reason, a reflexologist will always work on all the points in both of your feet. If you had a sinus problem, for example,

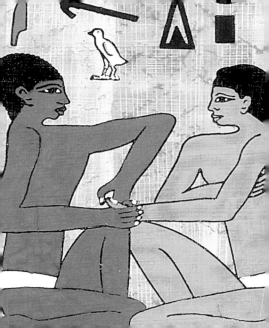

a good reflexologist would address it by manipulating both feet all over, not only the tips of your toes, where the sinus points lie.

In addition, some reflexologists manipulate the hands and ears, which are also believed to contain points that correspond with various body organs and systems. But most favor the feet, which have the following advantages over the body's other extremities:

Size: Because the feet are fairly large, their reflexology points are spread out enough to be worked on individually.

Sensitivity: The feet are rich in nerve endings; they contain even more of these sense receptors than the hands do.

Shape: Since they are similar in shape to the hands, they can be held and manipulated comfortably.

Neutrality: For most people, the

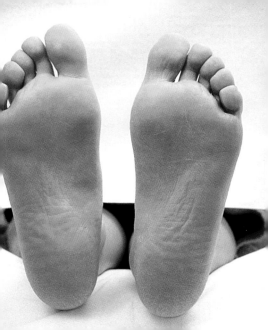

feet are a relatively "impersonal" area that a stranger can touch without violating their sense of personal space.

Need for tender, loving care: The feet work hard, supporting the body's weight and getting pounded day in and day out.

To get the most out of this therapy, you should put yourself in the expert hands of a trained reflexologist. You can find reflexologists in private practice in large cities, as well as on the staffs of many health clubs and spas.

You can even practice reflexology on yourself, although it's impossible to relax completely when working on your own feet. For the best results, bone up on the basics before you start by learning from an experienced reflexologist or a good manual.

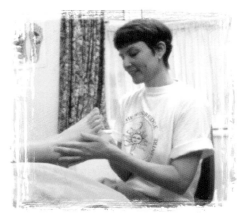

What to Expect in a Reflexology Session

A visit to a reflexologist may leave you feeling better physically and mentally. Your chronic minor aches and pains might fade or vanish temporarily. At the very least, you can expect a reflex-ology session to be a relaxing and pleasurable experience, creating a feeling of well-being.

You will most likely be lying faceup. The reflexologist might provide a special massage table or recliner for you to lie on, or simply ask you to lie on a bed or couch, with your feet all the way at its foot. Then she will position herself at your feet, sitting at a height that lets her work on them comfortably. She will cleanse your feet

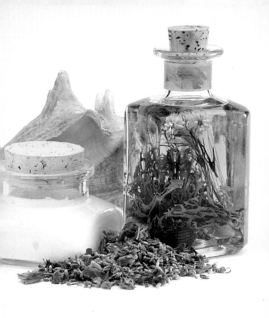

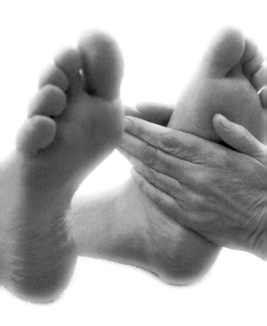

and may apply a small amount of cream or lotion to make the skin softer and more flexible. In addition, she might play soothing music or nature sounds, or work in silence, depending on which you find more relaxing.

A reflexologist will always work on both of your feet in the course of a session, for two reasons: first, some reflexology points are present on only one foot, so both feet must be manipulated to cover all the points; and second, organs that come in pairs, such as the kidneys, have two points, with the one on the left foot governing the left kidney, and the one on the right ruling the right kidney. The reflexologist works on one foot at a time, supporting it in one hand while manipulating it with the other. Although the core techniques of this discipline involve finger pressure on the various points in the foot, the practitioner may also use the palms, sides, and backs of the hands to stimulate these points and release tension.

Reflexologists use the hands and fingers in three basic techniques developed by Eunice Ingham:

Thumb-walking: With the palm facing down and the tip of the

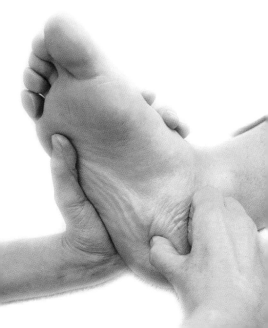

thumb touching the foot, the therapist flexes the first joint of the thumb to make the tip move, or "walk," along the area being worked. This technique is used on the fleshy areas on the sole of the foot, which can stand up to the motion of this relatively forceful pressure.

Finger-walking: The same procedure is followed as for thumb-walking, with the tip of the index

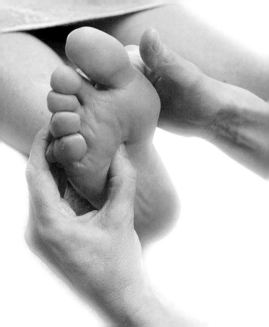

finger on the side facing the thumb doing the strolling. This technique is used on sensitive, bony areas of the foot that require a light touch.

Rotation on a point: While the thumb of one hand presses on a reflexology point, the other hand rotates the foot around the area being pressed. This technique is used on points that may be tender, as the rotating action distracts the subject from the pressure exerted by the thumb.

In addition to these techniques, the therapist might use a variation on the rotation technique: rotating the foot while thumb-walking, flexing the foot forward and backward, or employing a "hook and backup" movement in which the thumb is pressed on a small point and pulled slightly to the left or right. Experts also might gently stretch, bounce, or rock the entire foot or lower leg, although these broader motions are intended to loosen up the muscles in the area being worked on, not to make contact with specific reflexology points.

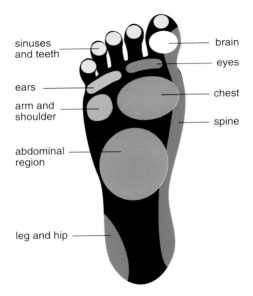

sinuses and teeth

brain

eyes

ears

chest

arm and shoulder

spine

abdominal region

leg and hip

Reading the Body Map on Your Feet

The body map on your feet is marked with numerous stops for the reflexologist's healing fingers—there are twenty-eight points in your toes alone!

Just as a map of this country is

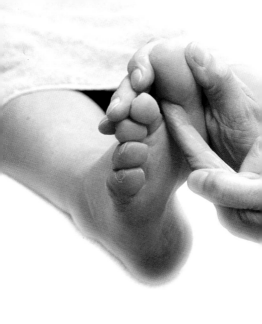

divided into states, the reflexology map is broken up into broad areas of the foot that correspond to large, general regions of the body. The head and neck area is governed by the toes; the chest, by the ball of the foot; the abdominal region, by the arch; the reproductive organs, by the ankle; the spine, by the inner edge of the foot; and the joints and muscles, by the outer edge of the foot.

The following section lists some regional points of interest on the reflexology map. (Remember that since you lie on your back in a reflexology session, your toes point up and your heels are down.)

Head and neck

Top of head, sinuses, and teeth: These areas are stimulated by working the reflexology points on

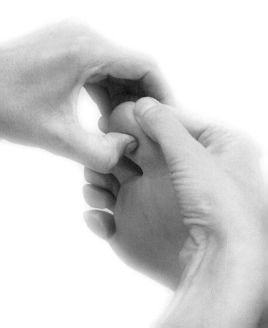

the tips of the toes. Such massage may prevent tension headaches and sinus congestion, and promote healthy teeth and gums.

Brain: The reflexology point assigned to the brain is on the sole of the big toe, just below the tip (toward the heel). On the left big toe, the point relates to the brain's left hemisphere, which rules the entire right side of the body, as well as language, mathematical and analytical ability, and logic. On the right big toe, it relates to the right hemisphere, which rules the left side of the body, as well as creative thinking, intuition, artistic ability, and spatial perception. Working this point on both toes may stimulate each type of mental energy and intellectual functioning.

Neck: The upper surface of the

base of the big toe is assigned to the neck. Working this area can ease the neck tension that typically builds up when you are under stress and unconsciously tighten the neck muscles.

Mouth: The band just below the toenail on the upper surface of the big toe governs the mouth. Manipulating this band encourages the salivary glands to produce saliva, which contains

enzymes that help begin the di-
gestive process.

Nose: Below the mouth area,
the next-lower band on the upper
surface of the big toe relates to
the nose. Rubbing and pressing
this point can relieve nasal congestion by improving circulation to
the nasal tissues.

Eyes: The bottom surfaces of
the second and third toes, below
the tips, contain the points that

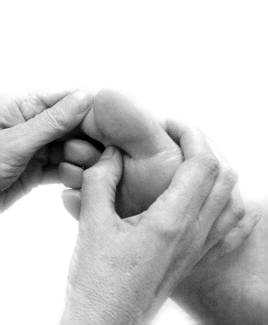

govern the eyes. Working them may reduce the strain that comes from doing close work or focusing for hours on a computer screen.

Ears: Right next door to the eye points, on the bottom surfaces of the fourth and fifth toes, below the tips, are the reflexology points for the ears. Massaging them may reward you with improved hearing.

Arms and legs

The points governing these limbs and joints are located on the outside of the foot.

Arm and shoulder: The reflexology points for the arm, including the shoulder and the elbow, are on the outer edge of the foot, between the fifth toe and the ball of the foot. Working this area relaxes the tension that can accu-

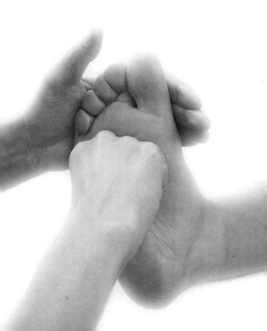

mulate in the arm muscles when carrying heavy loads.

Leg and hip: The leg, from hip joint to ankle, has its reflexology points in a triangular area on the outside of the foot between the arch and the heel. Rubbing this section can help relieve the stiffness that often comes from traveling or sitting too long at a desk.

Spine

The inner side of the foot, from the base of the nail on the big toe down to the beginning of the heel, corresponds with the spine. The side of the big toe contains the points for the neck vertebrae, and the remaining edge of the foot includes a long line of reflex points, one for each vertebra from the base of the neck all the way down

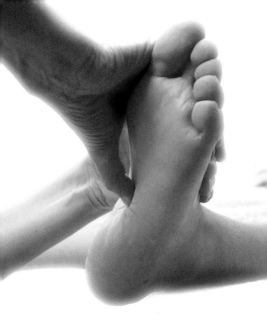

to the base of the spine. Manipulating these points may help keep
the spine loose and relaxed; it
may also improve posture as well.

Treating the Feet

Reflexologists turn to the hands when they want to treat the feet themselves. To affect the sole of the right foot, for example, the therapist works the right palm; for the top of the foot, the back of the hand; for the big toe, the thumb; for the other toes, the fingers; and for the ankle, the wrist.

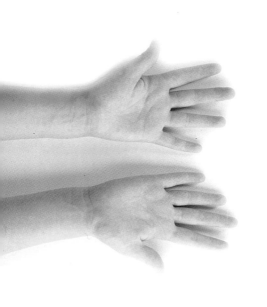

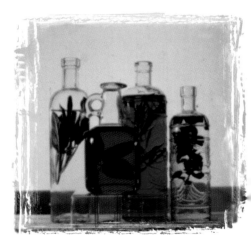

Alternative Healing in America Today

Eunice Ingham founded the first reflexology school in the United States in 1973. Since that time, this healing art has gradually moved from the fringe toward the mainstream. In recent years, interest in reflexology has risen dramatically, along with increased curiosity about all forms of alternative healing and preventive medicine. A variety of factors is responsible. These include:

• the increasing desire to deal with stress and its deleterious effects on physical and emotional health;

• the ever more technological and impersonal character of

modern life, which creates a more urgent need to seek human touch and heed the messages of one's own body;

• the desire to strengthen the immune system;

• the movement for health care reform and the American medical establishment's consequent appetite for low-cost, noninvasive methods of addressing the body's imbalances before they create pain and illness and require costly surgery or therapy.

Reflexology is often grouped with other therapies under the heading of "bodywork." Other popular forms of bodywork include:

Swedish massage—the stroking and kneading of muscles throughout the body to relieve tension (the type of massage with which Americans are most familiar).

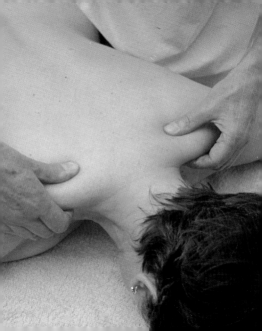

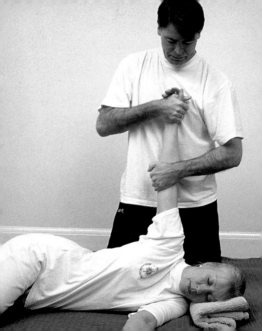

Shiatsu—applying pressure to selected energy points instead of stroking or rubbing.

Aromatherapy massage—pressing and stroking muscles using fragrant essential oils that penetrate the body.

Sports massage—deep-muscle rubbing that focuses on the body parts emphasized in a particular sport, such as the legs after bicycling.

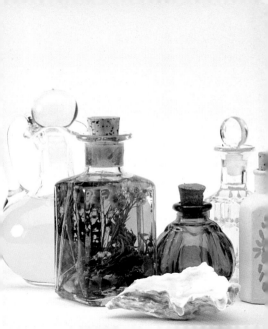

Therapeutic touch—placing the hands close to, but not on, the subject's body to increase relaxation and the flow of positive energy.

Little scientific research has been conducted on reflexology in the United States thus far, but a 1993 study demonstrated that this technique was able to reduce women's premenstrual syndrome (PMS) symptoms. The study's positive findings may lead to research on other ailments. Who knows what exciting powers reflexology might display in the next few years?

Meanwhile, Eunice Ingham's work is being carried on by her nephew, Dwight Byers, who directs the International Institute of Reflexology in Saint Petersburg, Florida. She would be surprised—and surely gratified—to see how

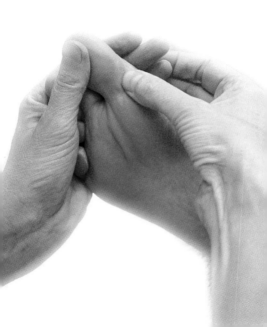

much interest the techniques she created and refined are generating today. In less than a century, modern reflexology has come a very long way.

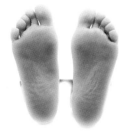

Notice:

If you have a medical problem, promptly consult your physician for advice.

The text of this book was set
in Futura Light at
Snap-Haus Graphics in
Edgewater, N.J.

Book design by
Snap-Haus Graphics